How To Get Arthritis Joint Pain, Stiffness and Swelling Relief for Dogs and Cats

The Best Way to Prevent and Treat Arthritis in Your Pets

Daniel Vang

Table of Contents

Chapter 1:
Introduction

I am a person who has loved animals since I was a little kid. As the eldest of two siblings, my sister grew up in a happy place with lots of family values, hard work, and lots of love.

Our parents taught us well, and we learned each day and the hard way. I witnessed my parents start from scratch and devote their lives to providing a good life for us.

They tried hard to build this little farm because it is their passion and dream. And as time went by, the tiny little farm became famous, and some tried to find us to buy livestock and all our products. People all over and out of town try to see us and continue patronizing us.

I love our way of life, but mostly I love all the animals we have. I grew up on a small farm with many livestock animals that my parents worked hard to attain. I even dreamed of becoming a veterinarian so that I could heal, tend to their needs, and take care of them. It gives me pleasure watching them every day.

It is our source of income, and I see my parent's commitment to it. We have different kinds of animals way back, and our parents make sure that we are well aware of all the things that go on our farm. They keep on teaching us many things and how to run them too.

We grew and sold vegetables and other root crops and, of course, Chicken, eggs, ducks, pigs, and we also sold cow's milk. So basically, I am a farm girl who loves our way of living, feeding the animals, helping my parents make money to support our needs, and our schooling, of course.

Despite my dream of becoming a veterinarian, I took a different path as I grew up a little older. I studied Business Administration and worked as a junior executive in a prominent office in the city. But the thought and feelings of loving animals never left me.

As my parents got old and my sister took a course on becoming a teacher, which she loves, our little farm was no more. We sold it, we moved and bought a small property in the city area which my parents adore. Both my parents passed away, and I live alone now.

I get lonely each day, and I feel alone going home. Sometimes I drain myself so that all I can do when I get home is sleep. I remember reminiscing about those days when my sister and I were still young and living on a farm full of love. Tending those animals makes me so happy and energized.

My interest in animals didn't go away, so I decided to purchase and take care of several dogs and cats. I love to go home every day. They mean everything to me.

I never got married nor had any children, so I devoted my life to taking care of all of them, whom I called my little angels. I ensure that they are well taken care of, giving them the proper nutrition, grooming them, and having their monthly check-up at the vet.

I admit it is a little costly, but it is all worth it. It is also a great responsibility because I live alone and have to leave my pets most of the time. Trying hard to tend to their needs and embracing being a parent fills the emptiness inside of me. I am once again the girl who lives on a farm that is very disciplined and very responsible.

I remember the day that I got Baeli, he was so adorable, and he took my breath away. He is the first dog that I got, and I am very fond of him.

He sleeps in my room like a company I didn't have because my sister lives in a different state and my parents died. He is very playful and loves to mess around all the time.

2

I am very observant, and I can easily detect something wrong, especially with my pets. The next day, I took the day off and took Baeli to the vet for a further check-up. He is fragile, and I can feel that he is in much pain.

He is a very active dog, and he rarely gets sick. He is always running and making some mess inside the house. He is the most mischievous one.

I was very anxious waiting for our turn because I wanted to know what was going on with my dog. I feel bad already that I thought I was not doing the best job as an owner. I keep blaming myself for this thing that happened, and to add, I felt I was not doing enough.

Finally, It is our turn. The vet asked me all the questions and what had happened for the past three days. All the necessary information like any accidents, food intake, or any falling? I told him that I only noticed it yesterday when I got home and I was alarmed, so I immediately scheduled it the next day.

He examined it and said that he must keep Baeli overnight for further observation. I got home apprehensive that I couldn't sleep. I have "What If's "in my mind. I keep blaming myself for whatever happens to my little angel, and I don't know if I can take it.

All of them are the reasons I got through my parent's death, and because of them, I regained strength and was able to laugh and be excited to go home after work.

I called my sister that night crying and telling her that Baeli was admitted. I cannot express how I feel to the extent that I was mumbling. She told me to calm down and assured me that everything was going to be ok.

She said that she would visit me this coming weekend, and I felt more relieved because I knew that she would keep me company even in a short time.

The clinic said that Baeli needed to be admitted for the next couple of days because he was dehydrated. They also informed me to visit the next day as the vet would discuss something important to me, which to my eagerness, I got there as soon as I finished work.

The vet told me that Baeli has a condition which is called "Osteoarthritis." Dogs usually have a specific underlying cause and are therefore often seen earlier in life. Underlying causes can include developmental disorders such as Hip Dysplasia or Cruciate Ligament Rupture and Injuries to the joint.

The vet asked me if he had undergone some accidents lately or if Baeli had fallen in high and dropped hard below. I don't know what to say because I know that Baeli loves to jump around the house and climb in high chairs. I felt terrible because I knew that I leave them the minute I went to work.

Although I am trying my best to be a good parent, tending to their needs, I am guilty of not being there most of the day. Now I am wondering when Baeli fell. I just can't imagine how hard it is.

The more the vet explained the condition of Baeli, I remembered the time when I was on the farm and how I was so cautious of our animals and pets during that time.

I was shocked because I didn't have a single clue about it. I never thought that this would happen to my precious dog. I cannot imagine what he must have felt and for how long; although the vet said it is good that it was caught early and can be treated, I am in agony knowing that my little angel is suffering and in pain.

He prescribed Baeli some pain relievers and told me to watch over and monitor his condition for the next three days.

4

The vet released Baeli and instructed me to take care of him for the next few days until he got back to his feet. I took a vacation to tend to him and all of them.

He can't walk that far for a couple of days, and I also have to give him full attention because of the drugs he was administered. The vet gave him the nonsteroidal anti-inflammatory drug. He said it could reduce pain and can decrease inflammation in the joints.

I took care of my little angel. He doesn't want to eat and is very restless, whining, and wants to cuddle with me the whole time. I am sad looking at Baeli suffering, and if only I can take it from him.

I can see that he is weak and doesn't want to eat or all he does is lay down the whole time. I am so sad and worried that I keep on calling my sister just to update her.

The next day was worsening, so I hurriedly brought him back to the clinic to be rechecked. Baeli was admitted again. The vet said that they would run more tests to make sure that the medications were working.

I went home feeling so devastated that I cried the whole night. The next day I went back there; the vet said he had changed Baeli's medication and advised me to send him into therapy.

He explained the situation of Baeli to me, and I must tend to all his needs and make sure that you must administer all medications at the right time. The vet also gave a list of healthy diets that Baeli must intake each day.

I was so sad, knowing that Baeli's situation might worsen if I didn't follow all the instructions, he gave me. I was also informed that there is no cure for Baeli's condition, but with all the proper medications and the weekly therapy, He can still recover and won't get into a life-threatening case.

I made sure that all the vet said was registered to my mind to give my little angel the best care that I could provide. As I held my little angel back to the car, I kept thinking about what I would do to keep him alive for a long time.

What will happen If I get back to work and nobody's home to tend to His needs. Driving a car with a lot in my mind and a heavy heart made me cry.

The next day, my sister arrived, and it was a relief that I could share my dilemma about Baeli's situation. We discuss it thoroughly to come up with solutions for His condition.

She volunteered to take Baeli with her. She said that she could look after him with great attention.

I know that I'm not too fond of the idea of being away with Baeli, but I don't have any reasonable choice. She said she would tend to all his needs because she works from home due to the Pandemic. I don't want to be impulsive, but without any doubt, I know deep in my heart that everything will be ok.

She spent the next two weeks with and tending to all Baeli's needs. I get back to work knowing that my sister is the best person to do my job with my little angels, especially Baeli. She was the one bringing her to therapy and making sure that I gave the medications on time.

I was so amazed that Baeli was improving so fast. The vet even said that the improvements were unbelievable. He said that to make sure that I watched Baeli's weight to help in the recovery.

The next few days were a little easier for me because my sister is there to help me tend to Baeli's needs and my other pets, of course, but it is also one of the hardest because she will get back to her place bring Baeli with her. The recovery is very remarkable, and I am happy about it. Changing the diet for Baeli did help a lot, and it keeps him fit and has much stamina.

The time has come that my sister must go home; Baeli is scheduled for a visit to the vet before bounding to his new home. The vet said to continue the therapy for another month, and it's a good thing that where my sister lives, they have a great facility there to cater to Baeli's treatment.

He also prescribes some medication so that if ever my sister notices that Baeli is in pain, she will give it to him, Vitamins to get him back on foot, and advice for a good diet and home exercise.

The next day, my sister is bound to go home. We also decided that she would take Hugo with them to keep Baeli company not to become sad. I was so sorry that after so many years and the thought of Baeli going away.

Although I know that He will be fine, it is the first time my little angel came into my life, It was hard saying goodbye, but I wish them well and know they are both going to be ok.

I went back to my routine, and I always see that the three angels are well cared for. I spend time with them over the weekends and make sure that I spend more quality time with them. I also hired a sitter three times a week to tend to them and walk them through maintaining their weight.

Choosing the right food, too, is in my best interest for my little angels. After what happened to Baeli, I am becoming more aware of all of them. I become more observant and keener to all of them. I am hands-on despite the busy schedules at work.

Regular check-ups are always my top priority, and I never miss a chance to check with them, especially during their grooming time. Baeli is having the time of his life with my sister.

With an expansive lawn and fresh air in the countryside, he is having fun.

Although it is a little slower, he is running again. My sister said that Hugo is a big help coming with them.

And to add more excitement to me, my little angels and I will be spending the holidays with them next month. I am already preparing for it and ensuring that my little angels will be very comfortable for a 5-hour drive.

I will hug and see Baeli and Hugo again and hope to bring them home when I get back.

Having them in my life makes it easier for me to get back after my parent's death.

Seeing Baeli suffer makes my heart bleed, and it hurts me more than I cannot do anything about it because I don't know what to do.

Now I am trying my best to be well informed, and I keep on researching this kind of disorder and some of the causes, symptoms, and all the home remedies I could find so that the next time this happens, I will know what to do.

I may be sound paranoid, but I know that prevention is better than healing.

It is a key to being well informed, and It is a must that you know all the information regarding it.

Having pets at home, we must be very observant and aware of what is going on. It is a great responsibility, but I tell you it is worth it.

Chapter 2:
What Causes Osteoarthritis in Animals?

Like humans, dogs are more likely to develop Osteoarthritis as my pets get a little older, with certain larger breeds- such as German Shepherds, Labrador Retrievers, Golden Retrievers, and Rottweilers- more prone to arthritis and decreased mobility.

Falling from height or being in a car during an automobile accident can also cause traumatic injuries that later develop Osteoarthritis.

While there are no direct causes for Osteoarthritis, underlying issues such as;

1) **Major Trauma**- specific causes such as dog attacks, another one can trigger trauma to them. Aside from being emotionally scarred from a traumatic event, most of them suffer from physical injuries too. They may have bone fractures that can cause arthritis later on as they get older.

2) **Hip or Elbow dysplasia**- Hip and elbow dysplasia are categorized as developmental disorders caused by dysmorphic and lax joint formation.

This malformation consequently results in abnormal wearing of bone over time, inducing the secondary development of Osteoarthritis and degenerative joint disease.

3) **Cruciate ligament injury**- The cruciate ligaments, in simple terms, are like two pieces of elastic solid that hold the knee together. If a cruciate ligament is damaged, the knee becomes wobbly and often painful.

The most common way the dog damages a cruciate ligament is by jumping, skidding, twisting, or turning awkwardly.

4) **Dislocation of the knee cap or shoulder**- It leaves dogs more vulnerable to developing arthritis. Typically, a dog with a dislocated kneecap will exhibit prolonged abnormal hindlimb movement, occasionally skipping or hindlimb lameness.

The dog will rarely feel pain or discomfort once the kneecap is out of position, only feeling pain at the moment the kneecap slides out of the thigh bone's ridges.

Most dogs who suffer and struggle with other health conditions such as Diabetes, Hyperlaxity, and Osteochondritis dissecans (OCD) may also be at a greater risk of developing joint arthritis.

Arthritis is a common health condition involving chronic inflammation in your joints. It causes pain and damage to joints, bones, and other body parts. There are some foods and beverages that add on to trigger these kinds of conditions. Research shows that dietary interventions, such as eliminating certain foods and drinks, may reduce symptoms and causes of Osteoarthritis in humans.

Many processed commercial dog foods contain grains such as wheat, rice, soy, which can cause your dog's blood sugar levels to fluctuate and increase pain. Limiting the grains of your dog's diet can decrease their inflammation.

Here are a few of our favorite "people foods "& dogs supplement for dogs with arthritis:

Whole food:

- Fiber-filled veggies: sweet potato, acorn squash, pumpkin
- Antioxidant-packed fruits: Blueberries, cherries, peeled apple, cantaloupe
- Vitamin-rich veggies: Broccoli, cauliflower, zucchini
- Leafy greens: Spinach, kale, collards
- Fatty fish: Salmon, mackerel, tuna, sardines

10

- Lean protein: Chicken, turkey

Oils:

- Omega-3 oils: Fish oil, green-lipped mussel oil
- Coconut oil (mix in with dogs food or use to sauté dogs veggies)
- Flaxseed oil (drizzle over dog's food)
- Herbs and spices
- Fresh ginger root
- Turmeric (fresh root or powdered)
- Cinnamon
- Parsley (bonus=breath freshener)

Certain foods and mineral vitamins can help humans as well as dogs. It can help prevent them from getting sick, and it can help them reach their bones more substantially.

Getting the right kind and balanced diet of protein, fat, and carbs, they'll get everything they need.

Dogs and cats will also get the essential minerals from there, including:

Protein: Dogs usually prefer foods high in proteins; at the same time, cats are descended from hunters, so they're natural carnivores. This is why protein is essential. It is where they get energy from their muscle repair, cells' growth, and body maintenance.

Animal-based proteins have all the essential amino acids pets need, including Arginine, Methionine, Histidine, Phenylalanine, Isoleucine, Threonine, Leucine, Tryptophan, Lysine, Valine, and Taurine.

Fats and Energy: Dietary fats come from animal fats or the oils of plant seeds. They're the most significant source of energy in your pet's diet.

They provide essential fatty acids, which dogs or cats do not make on their own. Fatty acids like Omega-3 can keep protecting their organs and insulate the body.

Carbohydrates: carbohydrates deliver energy, help maintain digestive health, and affect reproduction. Fiber is a type of carbohydrate that affects the bacteria in your pet's intestine.

Vitamins and Minerals: Dogs and Cats must need to get the right balance of vitamins and minerals every day. It will help them to get healthy and strong.

Here are some examples that you must include in your pet's daily needs.

Potassium- is an electrolyte vital to your dog's health—potassium aids in functioning electrical charges in the heart, nerves, and muscles.

Chlorine- according to CDC, Chlorinated water is safe for both Humans and Animals to drink in concentrations up to 4 milligrams per litre.

Iron- The daily recommended iron intake for adult dogs is 0.5mg/kg of body weight. The requirement is slightly higher for growing and nursing puppies since mothers' milk contains a low concentration of iron.

Copper- In health, copper plays a role in forming a dog's bones, connective tissue, collagen, and myelin (the protective covering of the nerves). Copper also helps the body absorb iron, making it an essential part of red blood cell function.

Zinc- This is an essential part of your dog's diet and contributes to them having healthy skin and fur. It is suitable for thyroid function and a healthy immune system.

Manganese- Dogs need manganese to produce energy, metabolize protein and carbohydrates, and make fatty acids. Manganese is an integral part of many enzymes and plays a role in maintaining bone and cartilage in joints.

Selenium: Selenium is a microelement which intake is essential for the correct function of the metabolism. In a dog's body, it is crucial, for example, for its anti-oxidant functions.

Iodine- Most iodine is used as an antibiotic in dogs. It is also used as an antibacterial for dogs and is very safe if swallowed.

Not having the proper nutrition, your pets might develop specific abnormalities in their bones that can cause arthritis.

They may get weak due to lack of all the nutrients they need and can also lead to weakness, and they can be prone to accidents such as falling.

In some cases, giving them too much can also lead to obesity. Most pets who do not exercise enough and eat unhealthy food are also a candidate for arthritis.

Giving your pets the necessary vitamins and minerals is a vital part of muscle and bone health.

Giving water must come to their diet too. About 60 to 70 percent of your pet's body is made of water. Without enough of it, your pet could get sick or die. Cats and Dogs have different thirst levels.

Dogs are thirstier when they're active, so make sure you have water for them as they exercise.

Giving the exact amount of all of this may help them experience this, and it will also prevent all the causes of arthritis. Knowledge is power. The more you are aware of what is best for your pets, the better.

Prevention is better than cure. So, the earlier that you are well aware of it, the better. There are so many ways to look for information, and you can search online or ask for professional help.

Nonsteroidal anti-inflammatory drugs (NSAIDs) play a significant role in controlling dog joint pain and inflammation.

Prescription medications such as; Galliprant, Carprofen, and Meloxicam are the safest options for controlling pain and inflammation compared to over-the-counter, non-veterinary products.

Chapter 3:
What are the Symptoms of Arthritis in Animals?

Osteoarthritis (OA), also known as a degenerative joint disease (DJD), is the most common form of arthritis in dogs. The condition causes progressive and permanent deterioration of a dog's joints, causing pain, stiffness, and lameness.

The most apparent symptoms of Osteoarthritis in dogs to watch out for are pain, stiffness, and lameness.

Often, stiffness and lameness are more noticeable after a dog has been resting, and the symptoms may start to ease or warm out as your dog moves around. Although this illness is most common to dogs, certain other animals like cattle may experience it too.

Other key symptoms to watch out for includes:

1) **Limping**- The action of walking with difficulty, typically because of a damaged or stiff leg or foot.
2) **Swollen joints**- Inflammation of the joints in dogs is simply another way of saying your dog is suffering from arthritis. It is a common problem in dogs, especially as they age or suffer an injury to a specific joint.
3) **Refusing to use the stairs or to jump into a car, or reluctance to move in general**- Like humans, dogs feel pain too. Most of them typically decreased the range of motion in the affected area of their legs.
4) **A noticeable change in behaviours, such as increased whining, irritability, or aggression**- Behaviour in humans if they don't feel good is like in pets. So, the more pain they or we think, the more irritable and they become mad. It is

15

very similar. They become grumpy, lose appetite, and have less activity.

5) **Restlessness, or seeming like they can't get comfortable**- The more pain the dogs feel, the more restless they are. It is like the cry for help that they are not feeling well. They are not comfortable. That's why they become agitated.

6) **Licking their joints**- They often lick the affected area to ease the pain or comfort themselves.

7) **Lack of enthusiasm for walks**- Dogs with Arthritis became limp and very reluctant to walk. Walking makes them feel more stressed because they feel uneasy and they feel pain.

8) **Shuffling when walking and failing to play usually**- Dogs who have joint pain walk by dragging one's feet along or without lifting them entirely from the ground. They also fail to perform their usual activities like playing.

Be on the lookout for these signs in your dogs. Always be observant. Having pets at home makes us happy, safe, and fulfilled, but if we can see that they are suffering and feel any amount of pain, we become worried and sad.

Being aware of our pet's condition is a must. Knowing what's going on in their body is our duty as the owner. We must be well informed, and we must have all the information that can give us all the ideas what to do if ever our beloved pets suffer from this kind of condition.

Always remember, they are like us too, we must take care of them. Knowing all the signs and symptoms of arthritis in our pets can help us determine if they are suffering from this kind of condition.

It is so much better than having all the information ahead of time because it is better than being ready if these things happen to our beloved pets. Most dogs and cats in their senior years have arthritis.

However, some dogs are more prone to arthritis than others: To name a few of this kind and their breeds.

Large breeds: These kinds of dogs, such as The English Mastiff, are some of the giant dogs in the world. As they age, they are more prone to developing arthritis.

Heavy dogs: Most dogs who are serious can acquire arthritis as they age too. According to some, medium breed dogs weigh from 35 to 65 pounds, and large and heavy are over 55 pounds. It is a common risk for developing arthritis.

Working dogs: A working dog is used to perform practical tasks instead of pet or companion dogs. The definition varies on an active dog; they are sometimes described as any dog trained for employment.

Athletic dogs: Primally bred to help humans hunt game, sports-hunting dogs such as retrievers, pointers, and spaniels are athletic and highly active.

Obese dogs: Obese dogs develop an increased risk for many types of cancer, diabetes mellitus, heart disease, and hypertension, Osteoarthritis, and faster degeneration of affected joints.

Dogs with diabetes: like humans, dogs may acquire this kind of disease. Most commonly to overweight people who don't exercise or those who don't love playing or walking around.

Cushing disease: Cushing disease is a severe health condition in dogs that occurs when the adrenal glands overproduce cortisol in the animal's body.

There are four stages of Osteoarthritis, both in humans and animals.

Both species may suffer this.

Stage 1- Pre- Osteoarthritis. Minor wear-and-tear in the joints. Little to no pain in the affected area. The preclinical stages, meaning the dogs are clinically normal.

Stage 2- Mild Osteoarthritis. More noticeable bone spurs. A dog's mobility is likely affected during some activities, such as playing fetch.

Stage 3 - Moderate Osteoarthritis. Cartilage in the affected area begins to erode.

Stage 4 - Severe Osteoarthritis. The patient is in much pain and should be given medical attention.

The Breakdown causes the bones to rub against each other, exposing your dog's small nerves and causing chronic joint pain. While Osteoarthritis is an unpleasant and painful condition, it's important to remember that it's widespread, affecting a quarter of all dogs at some point in their lives.

The symptoms of arthritis in dogs often start slowly and get worse over time. Dog parents may miss the early stages of the disease when their four-legged friends are experiencing only a tiny amount of discomfort.

Arthritis is a long-term condition that needs life-long management. Arthritis slowly worsens over time, but most dogs can live happily for many years after diagnosis if well managed.

Chapter 4:
How is Arthritis in Animals Treated?

What medicines can I give my dog for joint pain?

Unfortunately, there is no cure for Osteoarthritis. Treatments aim to allow pets to use the affected joint or joints without pain.

There is no single approach to treatment that is successful in every case, and most dogs and cats need a multi-modal approach, including:

Pain relief: Osteoarthritis can be painful, and so in some animals, long-term medication is needed. Although long-term medicines can have a risk of side effects, this risk must be balanced against pain from Osteoarthritis if the drug is not given.

Exercise: while exercise can cause discomfort in the short term, training is essential to keep your pets fit and healthy. There is no exact rule on how frequently they exercise.

Weight control: pets that are an ideal weight have fewer painful episodes and slower progression of Osteoarthritis than overweight animals.

Food supplements: glucosamine, chondroitin, and green-lipped mussel extract have been proposed to help treat Osteoarthritis. While the effect may not be dramatic, minor improvements may be seen.

Diet: diets containing omega 3-fatty acids may be a natural anti-inflammatory action that may help relieve discomfort associated with Osteoarthritis.

Therapy: physiotherapy and hydrotherapy are essential in the treatment of Osteoarthritis. It can build muscle, improve joint use, reduce muscle stiffness, and be good exercise. This therapy needs to be discussed carefully with your vet initially to avoid making painful joints worse.

Inflammation of the joints in dogs is simply another way of saying your dogs are suffering from arthritis. It is a common problem in dogs, especially as they age or suffer an injury to a specific joint. It may lead to this illness, and it can also make your dogs or cats suffer and be in pain and can also be life-threatening.

Observation of your Dog at home is a powerful diagnostic tool. Dogs rarely vocalize unless they are experiencing acute, sharp pain, so it's essential to monitor their habits and behaviour. Be mindful of your dog's condition, be observant, be aware of what's going on in your dog's everyday routine and behaviour.

How can I relieve my dog's joint pain naturally?

There are multiple causes of arthritis and chronic joint pains in dogs and cats, often in combination. If your pets have arthritis, there are several ways you can help them feel more comfortable every day.

Control weight and diet: Maintaining a healthy weight is essential to managing osteoarthritis joint pain in your pets. Make sure that they eat healthy and nutritious food every day. It is crucial to discuss your dog's weight with your vet and create a weight loss plan if needed.

Offer a soft bed: Usually, dogs don't need soft beds; they need to rest on a firm surface; they may have trouble getting into and out of it, especially if they are too old.

But in cases of a dog that feels pain and has Osteoarthritis, they must feel comfortable to ease their pain. It can make them calm and will have a good sleep.

Install ramps, cubes, and slip-free flooring: Use portable ramps or steps for places your dog can no longer jump. It can ease their pain, and it will be easier for them.

Try massage and exercise: You can gently massage your dog's sore spots to increase blood flow and apply alternating cold and hot compress in the affected area.

Make time for grooming: Grooming makes the dog relax. Through this, it can ease them from their suffering and the pain that they are experiencing.

Try Herbal Medications: You can choose alternative medications for your dogs. These kinds are primarily available anywhere that you can even buy them without prescriptions. One of the best examples is Kratom, it is an excellent herb for pain in your dog. It has a calming effect for anxious and restless dogs who are in pain. But always make sure that you have the correct information about it.

Non- medical support: Acupuncture is increasingly popular for treating canine joint pain and is beneficial for some dogs.

Hydrotherapy: Making your pets swim in a warm water pool or using an underwater treadmill is a great exercise that can improve muscle mass without overstressing joints. It can also help them relax and make them feel.

Anti-inflammatory medications, dietary supplements, and chondroprotective agents can treat Osteoarthritis.

The vet may prescribe nonsteroidal anti-inflammatory drugs to decrease inflammation, medications to reduce inflammation and pain. Chondroprotective agents such as Cartrophen help the body repair cartilage and stimulate its functions.

Home remedies such as "Turmeric "are also one of the best

home remedies for your pet's painful arthritis. As spice-rich in antioxidants, turmeric can help reduce inflammation and damage to your dog's joints.

The recommended amount based on your dog's weight is a perfect pain reliever and has anti-inflammatory properties.

Having all the correct information about this is much easier to treat your pets. Ask for professional help, or you can research your own. Tending to their needs and making sure that they are well taken care of may reduce the risk of the worst cases of arthritis.

Chapter 5:
What Types of Animals Get Arthritis?

Although arthritis may occur at any time, it is much more common in the later years of animals' life. The most common animals that usually get arthritis are dogs and cats. They are prone to these kinds of ailments. However, dogs are more likely to get arthritis than cats, but cats and other animals suffer from it.

Arthritis is rarely recognized during life in wild animals. Various alterations can be suspected in well-known joints, such as the wrist complex of the hyena or the shoulder complex of the felines.

An animal with arthritis may favor one or more of its limbs or have a distinct limp. The severity and limp will depend on the joints that are affected.

Limping is often more pronounced immediately after the animal wakes up from sleeping and becomes less pronounced as the animal begins moving.

Spondyloarthropathy is a painful arthritic affliction of humans that also occurs in wild mammals. Important questions remain concerning the underlying causes of spondyloarthropathy in mammals, mainly whether it is infectious in origin or driven by genetic predisposition and environmental stressors.

Different kinds of animals can also experience this, such as;

Dogs: Large breeds of dogs tend to have arthritis. It is most common in their later years and in those who have experienced physical trauma.

Cats: Cats may also be prone to arthritis, most especially obese ones.

Aquatic fish such as Dory Fish, zebrafish, and ray-finned

fish: Fish with synovial joints can get creaky. Thus, these fish are susceptible to arthritis.

Gorillas and other kinds of monkeys: Most large outbred rhesus monkeys can also acquire arthritis.

Elephants: If they are held captives and don't do much exercise, which can cause obesity and become lame, they are prone to developing bone and joint diseases such as arthritis.

Bears: Because of their prominent features and bones, they can also be prone to arthritis, especially in their later years, where they can no longer have the same activities.

Like humans, animals have bones too, so it is commonly known that as they get old.

Causing stiffness, swelling, and sometimes unbearable pain in affected joints, it involves many people in the world and animals.

Many people don't know that we're not the only species plagued with this debilitating condition, animals get arthritis too, and it's just as painful and distressing for them.

Most of them are neglected and abused, they have health conditions, and arthritis is one of the common issues that the animals have to deal with in their life span. It is sad to think about the animals that no one is taking care of them.

Imagine the pain and the suffering of these animals that don't have the luxury to have a veterinarian. Gladly there are so many volunteers and agencies, both local and international, who deal with these concerns; the only advocacy is to help animals without somebody to take care of them and those who suffer illness like this.

Here are some tips on how to take care of your Dogs and Cats;

1)   Provide a protective and clean-living environment for your pets.

2) Always keep fresh water available.
3) Feed a quality diet and prevent obesity.
4) Have your pet examined by a veterinarian regularly
5) Provide ample opportunities to exercise.
6) Parasite control and dental care, grooming

Conclusion

Having a horrible experience with one of my little angels is one of a person's greatest fears. Baeli is the most precious of them all, I did everything I could, but when the vet diagnosed Baeli, it felt like I was not doing enough.

I keep blaming myself for what happened to my precious angel; the thought that I could not answer all the questions that the vet was asking makes me feel bad.

I admit that before it happened, I thought I was doing the best I could on tending to all their needs, but I left them for work and went home to them thinking that what I was doing was enough.

I don't have any idea about arthritis and that dogs and cats can acquire them. I am clueless in these kinds of situations; the thought never crossed my mind. My guilt haunts me after what happened to Baeli, and the next thing I know is I become paranoid that this thing will happen to the rest of my angels.

The schedule of their monthly check-up was number one in my priority, the second was the diet must be as healthy and complete as possible, but always bear in mind that your pets may love to eat food fresh from your plate, but just because they like it doesn't mean it is good for them.

It made me aware of what might happen to my other pets. It gives me a more intense feeling that I have to check them once in a while. Being single and working, I can't bear that something might happen again while at work.

Those table scraps could lead to extra on your pets. More than half of all dogs and cats in the U.S are overweight and obese, which can also cause arthritis. They must consume High fiber foods at a minimum intake. Too much isn't suitable for young cats and dogs that are still growing.

Their energy needs are high, so their diet should have more fat and protein. We must try our best to find out legit information to be well informed.

Gathering the correct information on how to take care of our pets and the proper diet for them is the best thing to do.

Like humans, pets need their daily dose of nutritious food, enough exercise, and weekly grooming in their routine too.

As the owner, we should give them the best care ever. I know that some find it very expensive, that's why it is not a joke to have pets.

Like humans, pets are people too. They need their daily dose of vitamins and supplements. Giving them the best vitamins is the key to dogs and cats being healthy and not prone to Osteoarthritis.

The best vitamin for them is "Pet Bounce Multivitamin with Resveratrol, "which is the best. It has the right amount of essential vitamins and minerals to keep their bodies functioning at their best. It helps them improve their overall health.

Pet Bounce is complete, and it has a balanced multivitamin formulation made for your Cat and Dog.

It is fortified with Resveratrol, a powerful antioxidant chosen for its ability to improve your pet's health, and it can increase their vitality. It has an advanced formula created specifically to support their health and well-being.

And if our pets suffer from pain and swelling of arthritis just like we do, you can help them with Homeopathic ingredients, which have historically been used to help treat the symptoms of joint pain.

You can find it in "Pet Bounce Homeopathic Oral drops" It is the best relief for arthritis and joint pain of your pets.

The homeopathic ingredients in Pet Bounce are designed to be absorbed quickly into the bloodstream via the mouth tissues-so you can be sure your pets get the correct dose.

It works fast and is very reliable. It helps your pets with their discomfort and pain as quickly as you expected.

With an all-natural, plant-based homeopathic blend, it is designed to help alleviate the symptoms your pet might be suffering.

It is very safe because it has no side effects. It is also easy to administer; you are done without forcing your pets to swallow big tablets or capsules with a few drops.

Help your pets to enjoy a healthy and active life. If they have arthritis and joint pain, they can be as sad as humans, feeling down and restless. Assure them that they are well taken care of by making sure they don't feel any pain.

In addition to feeding and exercising your dogs and cats, other aspects of general care are needed to keep your dog healthy throughout its life. They also need mental stimulation and nurturing to thrive.

Providing these things is essential for keeping your dog healthy and safe and sets the foundation for a long, happy life for your beloved pet.

Giving the best care for your pets is a must. Providing a safe and comfortable home for them is your priority. It is like having your kids tend to their daily needs. They are family; they need tender loving care as well.

Although we know that it is a great responsibility, the feeling is gratifying for all its worth at the end of the day. It will bring happiness to you that money cannot buy.

To test whether your pet likes the product, here is a trial bottle of Pet Bounce

Multivitamin only through the link at https://bit.ly/beta99.

SCAN ME

www.ingramcontent.com/pod-product-compliance
Lightning Source LLC
Chambersburg PA
CBHW011034050426
42335CB00055B/2862